Mudras
Ancient Gestures to Ease Modern Stress

Mudras
Ancient Gestures to Ease Modern Stress

Emily Fuller Williams
Illustrated by Stuart Prado

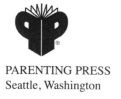

PARENTING PRESS
Seattle, Washington

Printed in the United States of America
Cover illustration and design by Julia Wharton
Line illustrations by Stuart Prado
Book design by Julia Wharton

Library of Congress Cataloging-in-Publication Data

Williams, Emily Fuller, 1946-
    Mudras : Ancient Gestures to Ease Modern Stress / by Emily Fuller Williams.
         p. cm.
    Includes bibliographical references and index.
    ISBN 978-0-943990-40-8
    1. Mudras (Hinduism) I. Title.
    RA781.7.W544 2011
    613.7'046–dc22
                                                    2010016332

Parenting Press
P.O. Box 75267
Seattle, Washington 98175

Visit us at www.ParentingPress.com to see more useful publications.

Foreword

As a psychologist, I spend my days with people who are frequently struggling to manage their emotions. Some are agitated and hyperaroused and come seeking calm. Some are lethargic and seek to find motivation and energy. Constant overstimulation from our technically complex lives has only made this problem worse. Meanwhile, on television wonder drugs promise a lifestyle of perfect balance.

How do we learn to manage strong emotional reactions? Researchers who study how children develop self-regulation find that it is related to the onset of language. Consider your own self-talk in an anxiety-provoking situation. "Stay calm. You'll be OK," we tell ourselves. Interestingly, newer studies have reported that the same regions of the brain that decode these linguistic messages are also important in interpreting wordless gestures. These wordless gestures may even be the starting point from which language developed. So when Emily first began to talk to me about mudras, it made sense that gestures could support our attempts to master our emotional responses.

Emily's work provides tools to manage our reactions at this older deeper level. With intuition that surpasses my left brain analysis, Emily works in a direct, physical, sensory manner to solve problems. I have incorporated her ideas into my work with great success.

Mudras: Ancient Gestures to Ease Modern Stress is the type of short, accessible book that can serve as a stimulus to learn self-regulation in a natural way. Emily presents the information in her typical straightforward manner, making the book easy to use at a moment's notice. I would heartily recommend this book as a tool for enriching your inner peace.

— Suzanne LeSure, Ph.D.
   CEO, Cornerstone Psychological Services
   Chair, Dept. of Psychology and Psychiatry, Medina General Hospital

Acknowledgments

The creation of this book has involved a great deal of growth and collaboration, and I am indebted to a number of people. To my husband, Robert Williams, for giving me the space and support to undertake this project, and for his editing and corrections work. To Elizabeth Crary for her help in structuring my material, and to Fred Crary for his technical expertise. To Heidi Nemeth and Jennifer Demitruk for their editing and corrections work.

To Amy Benza, Joyce Emrich, Suzanne LeSure, Ann Masternak, and Eve Whitmore, for opportunities they created to teach mudras and other stress reducing techniques to children and adults and for providing community outreach programs in which I taught mudras.

Friends who gave significant support were: Louise Grant, Alma Dancer, Debra Frantz, Barb Krecic, Natalie Kroman, Mary Kugel, Tammi Hanson, Rebecca Reynolds, and Laura Weldon.

Finally, this would not be the book it is without the field testers: thank you so much for your help.

Contents

Welcome

Hello. I'm pleased that you picked up my book.

You may have picked it up because you are curious about mudras or you may have a concern that impels you to want to change.

You may:
- parent a young child and need patience and energy
- be angry and need to release it so it doesn't consume you
- feel stressed and need to relax to avoid burnout
- be burdened with grief and sadness
- need a focused mind in order to study
- need to find a job to support yourself
- want more joy in your life

There is something magical about mudras. They have helped people with all the issues above.
They can help you as well. As a professional massage therapist and practioner of mudras, I know their power and I want to share it with you.

When you go to massage therapists, they use their hands to help you feel better. When you practice mudras, you use your own hands to feel better. That power to bring a sense of well-being is in your hands. This book will teach you how to use them.

You will need two things for mudras to work: motivation and commitment. Motivation to get started, and commitment to keep going. The investment in *you* will be worth it.

I wish you much success on your journey.

— Emily Fuller Williams

Part One:
Getting Started

Three stories about mudras
What are mudras and how can they help?
How long will I need to do mudras before I feel a change?
How can I get started with mudras?
I'm so busy and stressed. How can I ever make time for mudras?
If I have an issue, how do I know where to start?

Getting Started

Three stories about mudras

My friend Estelle was going to a family wedding. She asked, "Could you show me a mudra that would help me stay calm around the people who make me crazy?" I showed her the mudra for patience, where middle finger bends to thumb.

Later, she said, "When I do the patience mudra I can put my own feelings on a back burner and watch what is happening, without getting caught up in other people's dramas. Then the situation is easier to endure. By practicing this mudra in advance, I was prepared. Old family patterns didn't bother me so much!"

Marie came to me for massages after her husband died. She suffered great sadness when she tried to do things she and her husband had enjoyed together, like walking in the parks. I taught her the cheerfulness mudra to reduce her sadness. She practiced wrapping her fingers around her thumb.

On her next visit, Marie said, "I was an usher at a Cleveland Orchestra concert this week. I started to feel really sad because I had enjoyed concerts so much with my husband, and I missed him. I then thought to do the cheerfulness mudra. To my surprise, I immediately started to enjoy the concert."

Belinda had been having a tough time. She felt her life was unraveling, and she was overwhelmed by her chaotic thoughts. When I saw her crying one day, I offered to teach her a mudra that could help her feel better.

I chose the tranquility mudra to help her calm herself. After a couple of minutes, Belinda turned to me with a beautiful smile and said, "My thoughts were going round and round, but now they've stopped." Her demeanor had changed completely.

These are three examples of how mudras have helped people in their daily lives. Throughout this book you will find other stories, but first more about what mudras are and where they come from.

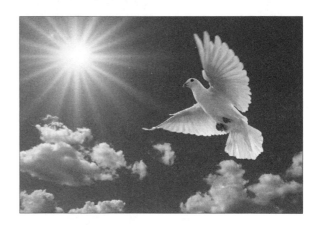

What are mudras and how can they help?

Mudras are hand gestures that impact energy. Mudras can change your feelings, your thoughts, and your life. Think of them as yoga for your hands.

What does *mudra* mean?

It comes from the Sanskrit language. I have seen it translated as "to seal" (as in sealing your intent, "this is how I want things to be"). It can also be translated as "that which brings delight" and "that which brings inner peace." All of these meanings imply that a change happens because of your active participation. You make a decision, and physically through your hands and your breathing allow something to happen.

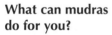

What can mudras do for you?

Your fingers can help you change your life.
You can use gestures to impact your inner responses. I do it, my clients do it, and you can, too. These simple gestures can affect how you habitually feel and think. By altering your actions a little, you can alter your life a lot!

Your fingers can help you impact your feelings.
Have you ever seen someone twirl her fingers in the air, as if she were screwing in a light bulb? When you feel anxious, this gesture can help you calm yourself.

Have you ever seen a child wiggle his hands at his ears? Or someone pull on his ears? Both gestures can help you release anger. When I pull on someone's ears as I give a massage, sometimes I feel like I'm letting out a windstorm of angry feelings!

Your fingers can help you change your thinking.
Have you ever seen someone play with his fingers, running the fingers of one hand up the other and back down while he's trying to study or understand something difficult? That playful gesture clears the mind, allowing you to think more clearly. Have you ever seen someone sit straight and tall, her whole being quiet, with her left hand over her right in her lap? She is using a powerful mudra to quiet her mind and body.

Why do people use mudras?

Because they work! A person may discover a mudra by accident or experimentation, but continue to use it because it is helpful.

Mudras are used in meditation practices because of their ability to calm the mind. They can be used to change our perceptions.

For example, when I practice the love mudra, I see more love in the world around me. Mudras can also be used to relax or energize us. They can help restore us when we feel underfed emotionally. In short, mudras allow us to practice self-care whenever we need it.

Why do mudras work?

There are several possibilities, but the simplest answer relates to the use of gestures. Before we talk, we learn to communicate with gestures. (Think of baby sign language.) Gestures have power just as sounds do. We can harness the power of gestures to move how we think and feel, just as we can use the power of sound to impact our energy and emotions.

For example, we use a lively march to pep us up, or Mozart to help us study. Movie makers rely on this phenomenon when they employ music to create moods in films. Gestures take us back to a basic level, our preverbal selves. Now, as then, we can create or alter our moods with gestures.

We can care for our inner selves much like a parent cares for a child. We can lovingly nurture ourselves through the use of gestures without waiting for someone else to do it for us.

Many people believe that mudras work because they affect how energy moves and is stored in the body. Some people are very aware of this energy and others not at all.

What does energy feel like?
This varies depending on the person and the mudra. Some people, when they do a mudra, report feeling:
• a sensation of heaviness in their hands
• a tingling in their fingertips or where the hands touch the body
• a decrease in the feeling of pressure in their stomach or solar plexus as energy leaves
• a warmth, or sensation of heat
• a calmness or quietness in their mind or head

How did mudras start?
They are thought to have developed out of natural gestures. The hand waving we teach a baby to say bye-bye looks like the mudra for letting go. Isn't waving good-bye a way of letting go? Many people put their hands over their chests when they feel distressed. This gesture is similar to the comfort mudra where you place your hands over your heart.

Where did mudras come from?
They have been used all over the world from ancient times. In the Far East they have been a part of dance and meditation for many centuries. Statues of gods and goddesses in mudra poses date from the 9th century in India. Ancient Egyptian friezes show royalty doing mudras. Christ was depicted on Byzantine icons using a mudra that Buddhists call the discussion gesture. To Hindus, this same mudra is the gesture of proclaiming a teaching.

No one knows for sure where the mudras originated, however, these natural gestures have been adopted by different cultures over many centuries. They predate organized religions as far as we know.

Do people ever discover mudras on their own?
Yes, they do! In fact, I call these "found mudras." When I teach mudras, frequently someone will say, "That's funny. I already do that." I've identified close to a dozen "found mudras" that we may be hardwired to do. We see an example of this self-discovery in the following story.

A therapist, who was working with a small boy, noticed one day that he was doing the patience mudra with both hands (middle finger touches thumb). She asked him, "Does the word mudra mean anything to you?" He said, "No." She said, "Why do you do that [the patience mudra] with your hands?" He said, "Because it makes me feel better. "

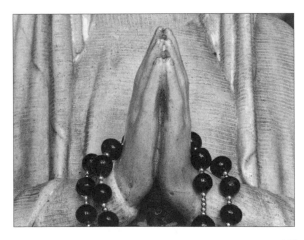

Who uses mudras today?

Kids, teenagers, parents, mystics, seekers, doctors, scientists, and practical people who want practical results use them. Teenagers are amazed when they can quiet their own minds. Parents are delighted to increase their energy and feel moments of calm. Practical people notice the ability to change their usual responses. For example, they are able to concentrate better when they lessen their anxiety.

If I start doing mudras, will I have to do them forever?

You may choose to do them forever, but you won't have to keep doing the same ones to get the benefits. When I have worked with one mudra for several months, I found all I needed to do was visualize myself doing the mudra, and I felt its effect. I achieved the benefits of the patience mudra, for example, just by imagining myself doing it.

✋ How long will I need to do mudras before I feel a change?

It varies dramatically from person to person, and even from mudra to mudra. It can be a couple of minutes or a couple of weeks. Sometimes you may not feel the effect even though it is working.

Some people feel the effects immediately.

I often teach the calming mudra first, because many people can feel tension leaving their fingers just after doing this mudra. Other people don't feel energy, so it will take them longer to notice the effects.

Sometimes a change occurs and you don't know it.

I feel something immediately with every mudra that I use, but it still takes me some time to notice if the mudra is affecting the rest of my life. So, a mudra may be working without our immediately noticing it.

I started doing the contentment mudra every day after a period of unrest. About two weeks later, someone mentioned how together and calm I looked. It was true I was feeling much more content, but I hadn't realized it until someone else observed it.

Sometimes people need to return to a mudra.

When I began to do the patience mudra, I did it regularly several times a day. When I became more patient, I stopped doing it. Now if I notice that I'm getting really impatient (especially at stoplights), I start doing the patience mudra again. I stop doing it when I no longer feel impatient. Mudras can be like tools – you pick the one you need, when you need it.

Mudras can change your perceptions.

Feeling like I lacked resources, I started doing the prosperity mudra. After a couple of weeks, I realized that my perception of my need had changed. Prosperity for me was no longer about grabbing and holding onto wealth, but rather about giving and receiving. Prosperity is really about being in the flow, where you know you have something worth sharing with others, and they in turn will give something back to you. The prosperity mudra helped me perceive this, and it changed my belief.

✋ How can I get started with mudras?

There are two different approaches to mudras. Do you need a random, creative, playful approach to really get yourself flowing? Or do you need a step-by-step, structured approach? Which one works best with your personal style?

Random, creative, playful approach

You could open the mudra section of this book randomly and start with that mudra or choose a number between one and twenty-four and do that one. If you find a mudra you are drawn to, you can begin with that gesture. If you find a mudra that is very hard, you can work with it until it is easier.

Another playful, random approach would be to use a die. The mudras in this book are organized into six categories. The throw of the die would determine which category to pick a mudra from. You could start with the first mudra in the category because it will usually be the easiest to do. If it doesn't resonate with you, try another in the category.

You can also mix up the way you choose mudras. You might want to do the mudras with a friend, playing with them. Try different positions when doing the mudras. I have done mudras with my hands on my head or my feet up on the bed. I have done mudras by candlelight, to the sound of ocean waves, and with my cat. I have done mudras visualizing silly things, like M&Ms flowing into my hands. Trying mudras in different ways can have some unexpected results.

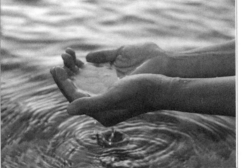

One evening a friend and I played with the self-confidence mudra for half an hour. We did it with our hands in many different places on the top of our heads, to our right, to our left, on our knees. We did it every way we could think of.

The next day, I started my taxes and found I could remember every detail I needed to know. I didn't have to look up a thing. I don't normally have much confidence in my memory, but that day I did!

Playfulness helps me; it doesn't help everyone. Use this approach if it works best for you.

Step-by-step, structured approach
Open this book to the beginning of the mudra section. Start with the first mudra. You can sequentially try a different mudra every night until you find one that really grabs you, or one that is really hard for you to do. If it is hard for you to do, it may be one that you really need.

You could look at the mudra wheel (see page 67) and choose a category, such as *release*, and work your way through it. Decide which one of the four mudras in that category works best for you, and then go on to the next category. When you work your way around the whole wheel, you will have chosen six mudras to do. Then, when you need a mudra from any of the categories, you'll already know one.

An alternate structured approach is to do one mudra from each category. When you've gone through the six categories, you start a second pass around the wheel, going to the second mudra in a category (but only if the first one didn't resonate with you).

Last, you could also ask friends what mudra you need the most. My friends all voted for the patience mudra for me. Friends who tell you the unvarnished truth are a great source of information.

I'm so busy and stressed. How can I ever make time for mudras?
There are several ways you can incorporate mudras into your life. You can use "found" time that would otherwise be wasted, or use "trigger" time in response to an event. You can structure regular time for mudras, if you work best with routines. Or you can use "reminder" time, where you have set up prompts or cues for yourself to help you remember to do mudras. Here are examples of each.

Found Time: Time that you would otherwise waste.
- Sitting at a stoplight
- Standing in a check-out line
- Sitting in a car as a passenger
- Waiting on hold on the phone
- Sitting in a meeting

Trigger Time: Time when you are (or may be) irritated or upset about something. For example, if you are distracted by two co-workers who are arguing, you can do a mudra. Other examples of trigger time are:

- While having a meltdown
- While watching your child have a meltdown
- When noticing you are getting stressed
- When studying and your concentration has lapsed
- When feeling fatigued or burned out
- When feeling like your perceptions are getting in your way
- When feeling frustrated or angry
- When feeling sad, lonely, or anxious
- Any time you feel like you need an attitude adjustment

Structured Time: Time you deliberately schedule to do mudras. Structure can be a time of day or related to an activity. For example:

- While still in bed in the morning
- After brushing your teeth
- While your baby takes a nap
- While taking a break at work
- Just as you get home from work
- After finishing dinner
- When studying or beginning mental work
- Right before going to bed

Reminder Time: Time associated with a cue or prompt that you set up for yourself. For example:

- When you notice the mudra book on the night stand
- When you see a mudra picture attached to the mirror
- When you hear the reminder message on the phone

How long does it take to do mudras?

Not long – about as long as it takes to play a piece of contemporary music. I suggest people do a mudra for two to three minutes. However, if you immediately get a sense of the movement of energy, you don't need to do it for much longer. Part of what you are waiting for is the feeling of movement. The effect of the mudra continues to work after you stop. For example, if my fingers tingle when I do a mudra, they continue to tingle after I stop.

If you don't feel the movement of energy, don't worry. The mudra may still be working. Some people are simply more sensitive to the movement of energy than others, just as some are more sensitive to light or sound. You may stop after three minutes.

If I have an issue, how do I know where to start?

Each of the twenty-four mudras fits into one of the six groups, four mudras in each group, as you can see in the table on page 21.

Mudras in Each Group		
Release	**Relax**	**Restore**
Calmness	Tranquility	Comfort
Release chaos	Patience	Contentment
Tension buster	Trust	Love
Release intense feelings	Self-forgiveness	Happiness
Recharge	**Reframe thinking**	**Refresh mind**
Energy	Prosperity	Balance
Replenish	Courage	Memory
Cheerfulness	Vision	Clarity
Self-confidence	Overcome obstacles	Focus

Do you want to nurture yourself, energize yourself, change your thinking, or refresh your mind? These translate to restore, recharge, reframe thinking, or refresh mind on the mudra wheel. Start where you feel the greatest need. Then what is your next greatest need? You are on your way!

When you are thinking about combining mudras, do release and relax mudras first. When you are not overflowing with feelings and are relaxed, it's easier to decide what to do next.

How can I remember to do the mudras?

As with many endeavors, a written plan can help you put your wishes into actions. Making plans can be unsettling to those of us who like a spontaneous approach. I'll show you how to make a plan.

First, envision what you want. To do that, create an image of what you want, and then make a goal with a measurable objective and a deadline.

Next, think about what steps are needed to accomplish your goal. These become your supporting or mini-goals. Then list what you need to do for you mini-goals. This becomes your "shopping list" or action items.

Last, finish the plan by choosing a date to review and revise it if need be, deciding how you will celebrate your success. Celebration is like positive self-talk, except it's an action honoring yourself. It will help keep you motivated. An example of a plan appears on page 22.

Aren't using mudras a lot like doing yoga?

Yes! Sometimes people call mudras "yoga for your hands." There are similarities and differences. Both mudras and yoga involve your breath and your awareness. Sometimes a mudra is part of a yoga posture. The mudras in this book use only the arms and fingers. Yoga involves stretching the body, making the body both flexible and strong. Mudras instead influence how you feel and think. Mudras are quick, simple, and portable. Only your hands need to be free. I invite you to try the mudras in this book. All you have to lose is some tension and stress.

We have looked at what mudras are, how they affect some people, where they come from, and how you can fit them into your life. In the next section, we will look at how to do each of the twenty-four mudras.

Plan	
Step	**Action**
1. Envision what you want. Imagine you are in the future. Describe how you want things to be.	*I want to sleep better at night.*
2. Make a personal goal that is specific and measurable.	*I want to sleep seven straight hours a night by March 15.*
3. Clarify mini-goals so you know what things you need to do to achieve your personal goal.	• *I will use the patience mudra every night for a week.* • *I will drink chamomile tea each night.* • *I will smell lavender each evening before bed.*
4. Establish action items.	• *I will put the patience mudra card by the bed.* • *I will buy lavender lotion and chamomile tea by Saturday.* • *I will put a pretty cup and the tea on a tray on top of the refrigerator so it is ready to go on Saturday.*
5. Date to evaluate	*March 1.*
6. Celebration plan	*I will rent a video of "Sleepless in Seattle" and watch it with a friend.*

Part Two
Using Individual Mudras

List of mudras by groups
Release • Relax • Restore
Recharge • Reframe thinking • Refresh mind

Using Individual Mudras

Through simple hand movements you can change how you think and feel

True peace and contentment ultimately come from within.
Mudras – simple hand movements – affect how feelings move through your body. With mudras you can allow feelings of contentment, happiness, and trust within yourself.

Mudras are a simple way to modify feelings.
When you release feelings that are stuck (anxiety, depression, fear, anger), you can express new feelings of trust, calmness, and abundance.

Different people experience mudras differently.
Try a mudra for 3 minutes. You may want to increase or decrease the time depending on how you feel when you do it.

The mudras are organized by groups: release, relax, restore, recharge, reframe thinking, and refresh mind. These are based on the functions of massage. Within each group, the mudras are organized from simple to more complex. The simpler ones use large muscles and large motions. The complex ones require more coordination because they use smaller muscles and finer motions.

The illustrations show the mudras as you would see them if you were facing someone who is doing them.

List of mudras by group

Release
Calmness – release anxiety
Release chaos – calm your mind
Tension buster – draw tension from the jaw
Release intense feelings – create lightness

Relax
Tranquility – create calmness and strength
Patience – accept life's natural rhythm
Trust – increase confidence and feel safe
Self-forgiveness – release guilt

Restore
Comfort – help with loss and grief
Contentment – increase current serenity
Love – stimulate love from within
Happiness – savor life

Recharge
Energy – recharge yourself
Replenish – fill up with energy
Cheerfulness – chase away sadness
Self-confidence – project positive energy

Reframe thinking
Prosperity – live with abundance
Courage – release fear
Vision – clarify dreams and needs
Overcome obstacles – open the way for positive energy

Refresh mind
Balance – reduce stress
Memory – increase mental power
Clarity – make clear decisions
Focus – increase calm and concentration

Release group

1 Calmness: Release anxiety

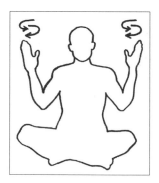

I taught this mudra to a Chamber of Commerce group. Later, a man who had been at that meeting told me he had taught it to a group of women in a prison. One woman thanked him and said she had felt something really ugly leave her arm when she did it. Sometimes we carry really heavy angry feelings in our arms, and the calmness mudra can help us let them go.

This mudra draws anxiety and tension to your hands and lets it drain out of your body.

How to do it:
- Sit straight and tall.
- Bend your elbows so your forearms are upright and hands are at ear level.
- Extend your fingers straight up, and rotate your hands back and forth at the wrists, as if you were screwing in a light bulb.
- Breathe deeply and slowly for 3 minutes as you rotate your hands.
- When done, let anxiety drain out by dropping your hands loosely to your sides and gently wiggling them.

Special note:
This and other mudras help release anxiety that many of us hold in the forearm area. Brush your arms with your hands as if to send those feelings away.

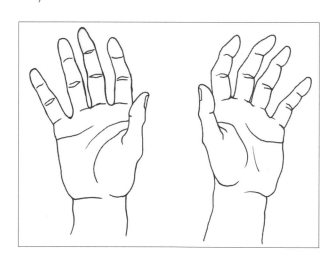

2 Release Chaos: Calm your mind

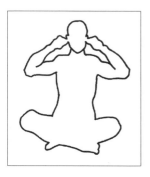

Cheryl never seemed angry. When giving her a massage, I never found anger any-where in her body. She told me she frequently pulled gently on her ear lobes for sustained periods of time. She just thought it was something she did to keep herself occupied. I think she was releasing anger when she did it, and that's why she was carrying so little around.

When you pull on your ear lobes, this mudra releases irritation and tension in your head. It is one of the ways to let go of thoughts that are going round and round.

How to do it:
- Sit straight and tall.
- Raise your hands to ear level.
- Grasp your ear lobe with your thumb and middle finger.
- Pull gently out and down a little.
- Breathe slowly and deeply for 3 minutes as you hold your ear lobes.
- Shake out your hands when you are finished.

Special note:
If my thumb and middle finger start to tingle, I know I'm pulling something out.

This mudra helps you let go of stress that you hold in your head, neck, and shoulders. People with headaches often respond well to this mudra. I believe it releases some of their anger. For years I've been pulling on people's ears while giving massages. Now I suggest they do it themselves.

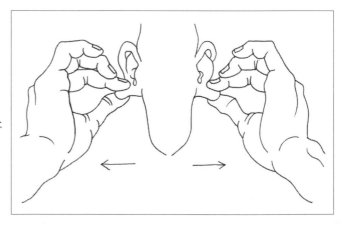

3 Tension Buster: Draw tension from the jaw

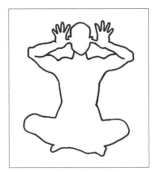

Janala came to me with jaw pain. She had also had a recent death in her family. I did release work on her body, and then I taught her this mudra. She felt really silly doing it. But she found she could relieve some of the pain herself, by imagining her fingers as antennae that released stuck feelings from her jaw when she breathed out.

Stresses of life often build up in your face and jaw. This mudra helps you release those tensions.

How to do it:
- Sit straight and tall.
- Raise your hands to ear level.
- Put your thumbs in the little hollow just in front of your ear canal.
  You will know you are in the right place when your thumbs wiggle as you open and close your mouth.
- Spread your fingers and imagine your tension radiating from your finger tips.
- Breathe deeply and slowly for 3 minutes.
- Lower your hands and shake them out when you are done.

Special note:
Try this with your thumbs touching your face and then not touching your face.

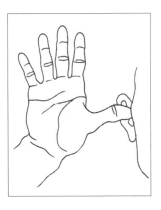

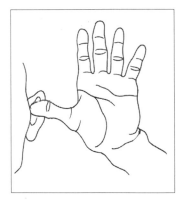

4 Release intense feelings: Create lightness

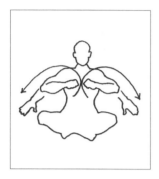

I taught this over the phone to a friend, Teresa, when someone she knew died unexpectedly. She said it really brought her relief. It didn't take away all the pain, but she felt lighter and more able to function.

This mudra releases heavy or fiery feelings and leaves you feeling lighter and more open.

How to do it:
- Sit straight and tall.
- Place your hands below your ribs at the midline of your body.
- While breathing in, make a grabbing motion as if picking up feelings, then move your hands to your sides.
- While breathing out, flick your hands down and out to the side to release the feelings.
- Repeat as needed.

Special note:
When you flick your hands down and out to the side, make sure no other person is so close to you that you are flicking your feelings onto them.

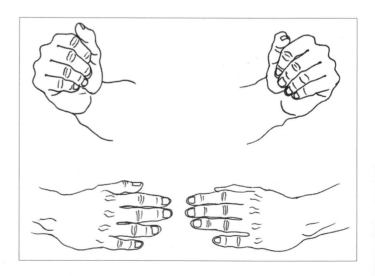

5 Tranquility: Create calmness and strength

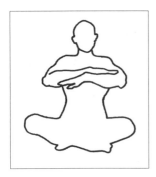

Louisa had a chronic intestinal disease. She was amazed at how much massage changed how she felt. One day she asked me, "How can I get the same feelings I get on your table when I'm not there?" This mudra flashed through my mind, and I taught it to her. She said, "I feel grounded and my mind is quiet. I feel like I am gently cradling a baby in my arms, and the baby is myself."

When you reduce the chatter of your mind you can focus and attend more easily.

How to do it:
- Sit straight and tall.
- Keep fingers straight.
- Place your right hand on your left forearm and your left hand under your right forearm, palms down.
- Breathe deeply and slowly for 3 minutes.

Special note:
One client said that the tranquility mudra worked for whatever was troubling her. For left handers, the tranquility mudra may be more powerful if the left forearm is on top of the right.

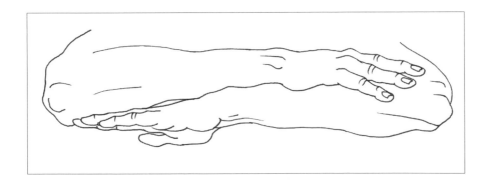

6 Patience: Accept life's natural rhythm

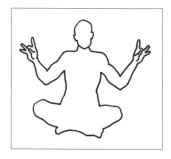

Emma had a deck of my mudra cards. When she had challenges, she would sort through the deck and choose a mudra to help herself. She chose the patience mudra when her mother was dying. She said, "I would sit down in a chair and do the patience mudra when all my worries would come flooding in. It helped. It really did."

Patience involves putting aside distractions. This mudra sends calming energy to your nerves and encourages patience.

How to do it:
- Sit straight and tall.
- Put your hands to the sides at ear level, palms facing forward.
- Make a circle with the tips of your thumb and middle finger. Keep other fingers straight up. Do this with both hands.
- Breathe deeply and slowly for 3 minutes.

Special note:
The patience mudra helps you be less attached to a specific outcome. You can watch what is happening without reacting thoughtlessly.

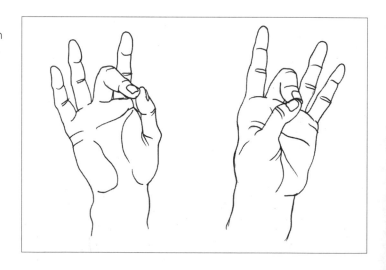

7 Trust: Increase confidence and feel safe

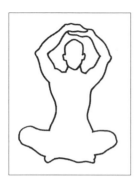

Sheila was a very quiet, shy person. She had experienced physical abuse when she was a child. A therapist sent her to me. Being touched safely and in a nurturing way changed her. Something that had withered in her came alive again. I taught her the trust mudra. She said she did her mudra in bed at the end of the day, and it helped her feel safe.

Many life experiences invite fear. When we are fearful we cannot respond to life's many kind offers. This mudra gives you a sense of safety and increases your ability to see and absorb good things.

How to do it:
- Sit straight and tall.
- Make a circle with your arms above your head, palms facing down. For women put your right palm over your left hand. For men put your left palm over your right hand.
- Think of yourself as being in a circle of safety.
- Breathe slowly and deeply for 3 minutes.

Special note:
As a left hander, this works better for me when the left palm is over the right hand.

Several people have told me they find this hard to do. They say they feel so exposed when they do it. If this happens, reverse your hands or do the mudra in a place where you feel safe.

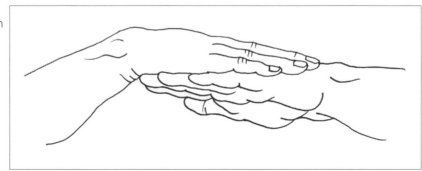

8 Self-forgiveness: Release guilt

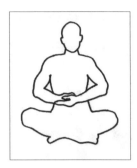

May came to me when she was feeling disappointed in herself. She said, "I'm not as strong as I thought I was. I had a roommate who was encouraging me to do really dumb things. I couldn't seem to stop myself while I was with her. So I moved out and away from her."

We did the mudra together at the end of her massage. She visibly relaxed while doing it. I was reminded again that forgiveness is not a thought. It's an act that we do; a conscious letting go.

Negative past experiences can block us from a happy life. When we let go of guilt and forgive ourselves we become open to enjoyment.

How to do it:
• Sit straight and tall.
• Rest your hands comfortably on your belly, palms facing up, with the fingers of your right hand in the palm of your left hand, thumbs touching.
• Breathe in forgiveness. Breathe out guilty feelings. Imagine them flowing out your right arm. Do this while breathing deeply and slowly for 3 minutes.

Special note:
Imagine your guilty feelings sliding down your right arm and out your fingers. When you are finished shake out your hands.

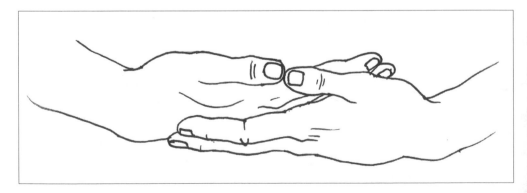

9 Comfort: Help with loss and grief

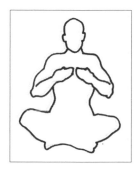

Ann had a life-threatening illness. She said it was often hard to find the energy to come in for a massage. I would use ginger lotion, and massage gently behind her ears, because I knew it comforted her. Once we did this mudra together before her massage, and she said, "I come here, and you teach me a mudra, and I feel so much better before I even get on the table!"

Life deals many losses – death of a parent, partner, or pet, also loss of job or dream. These losses leave your heart feeling depleted. This mudra helps you nurture your heart.

How to do it:
- Sit straight and tall.
- Put your hands on your chest, fingers pointing towards each other.
- Imagine your hands warming your heart.
- Breathe deeply and slowly for 3 minutes.

Special note:
If you feel too much energy or your heart races, lace your fingers together.

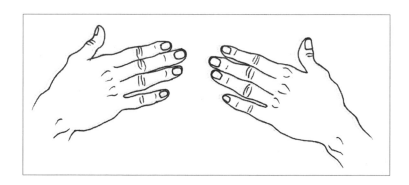

10 Contentment: Increase current serenity

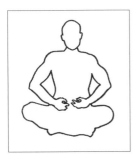

Cassie had many fears remaining from her childhood. When I massaged her, she was able to release some of her fear. I tried teaching her a mudra for fearlessness, and this is what she said. "The contentment mudra helps me more, because what I fear is a loss of connection. When I do the contentment mudra, with my fingers interconnected, I feel connected right away, and my fear disappears!"

Contentment feels as if you're having a nice cup of tea with a friend. You quit worrying about the past and future and are totally mindful of the present.

How to do it:
- Sit straight and tall.
- Hold your hands a few inches apart above your lap.
- Make a circle with the thumb and middle finger of the right hand. Make another circle with the thumb and little finger of the left hand. Relax your other fingers. (For men, switch hands.)
- Breathe deeply and slowly for 3 minutes or however long seems natural. When you are finished, shake out your hands.

Special note:
The contentment mudra is one of my personal favorites. You can use this mudra as an antidote to irritation, frustration, or other unsettling feelings. Practicing this mudra brings you into the present moment, leaving irritations and frustrations behind. If for you, contentment is about relationships, interlock the circles made by your two hands.

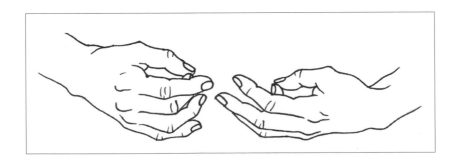

Restore group

11 Love: Stimulate love from within

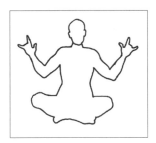

Agnes lived by herself and sometimes felt isolated and lonely. She really loved massage because then she didn't feel lonely. I suggested this mudra for self-care. Agnes agreed to do it every day for one month. Afterward, she said, "It was odd, because I became more aware of love. When someone acted loving toward me, I was much more likely to notice it, and I felt loved. I also saw more love in the world."

Love is the glue that holds us together. It starts with self-love. When we love ourselves, we have love to share with others.

How to do it:
- Sit straight and tall.
- Bend your elbows and raise your hands to shoulder level.
- Curl your middle and ring fingers down into your palm while extending your thumbs and other fingers.
- Breathe deeply and slowly for 3 minutes.

Special note:
In American Sign Language this sign means "I love you." When your palms are facing out, you are sending your love out into the world. When you turn your palms toward yourself, you are nurturing yourself with love. When I demonstrate this mudra the palms of my hands are usually facing away from from me; however, I'm told by others that they feel the impact of this mudra more if they turn their palms to face themselves. Try this mudra several ways. First, put your hands in front of you, with your palms facing out. Then, turn your hands so that you are looking at your palms. Finally, put your hands on either side of your head, with your palms facing you. Which works best for you?

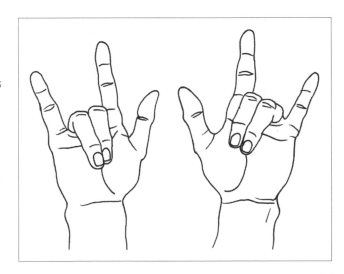

12 Happiness: Savor life

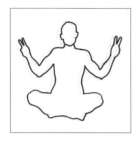

Raphine said, "When I do this mudra, it reminds me of the peace sign of the sixties. That makes me laugh. I feel silly and I lighten up. When I lighten up, I feel more connected to my silly, creative side. That makes me feel happy!"

Happiness comes from within. This mudra helps you find a place of joy within yourself.

How to do it:
- Sit straight and tall.
- Raise your hands to shoulder level, with palms facing forward and your fingers straight up.
- Bend your ring and little fingers in to touch your palms. Wrap your thumbs around them.
- Breathe deeply and slowly for 3 minutes.

Special note:
This mudra grants you permission to be light, silly, and playful. This kind of energy connects you to your natural creativity.

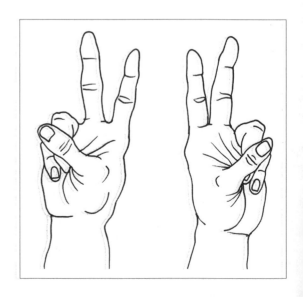

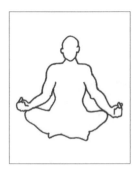

Recharge group

13 Energy: Recharge yourself

Angela, the parent of two small, very active children, complained of exhaustion so I taught her the energy mudra. The next week, Angela said, "When I go into a quiet, dimly lit room for just a couple of minutes and do this mudra, I feel plugged into a peaceful energy source. When I walk out, I feel much more able to handle things."

Children need constant attention, guidance, and patience. Parents can feel overwhelmed. Whether a parent or a person with a busy schedule, recharging yourself can do wonders for your ability to cope with a situation.

How to do it:
• Sit straight and tall.
• Rest your arms at your sides.
• With palms upward, make circles with the tips of the thumbs and index fingers.
• Breathe deeply and slowly for 3 minutes.

Special note:
The energy mudra plugs you into the wall socket of life. If this mudra doesn't work for you, try the replenish mudra.

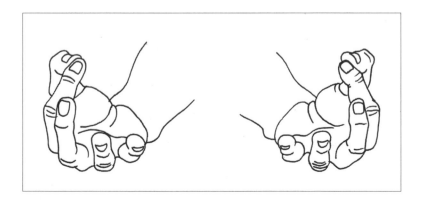

14 Replenish: Fill up with energy

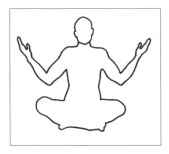

Elaine was 39 years old and the mother of three small children. She said that she never had enough energy because she was constantly on the go. Elaine added that she had trouble taking time for herself, and she really needed someone to take care of her. I suggested the replenish mudra when she needed a quick energy boost. She left smiling, and she continues to use this mudra when her energy level lags.

This mudra counters fatigue and lethargy. This is the mudra I would suggest when you feel like your battery is low.

How to do it:
- Sit straight and tall.
- Put your arms out, elbows down, palms up, so you look like a W.
- Fingers are extended straight out from your wrists and are touching each other.
- Imagine energy collecting in your hands and arms and flowing into your body.
- Breathe deeply and slowly for 3 minutes.

Special note:
This mudra feels natural outside in the sunshine.

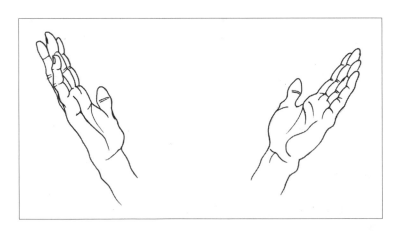

15 Cheerfulness: Chase away sadness

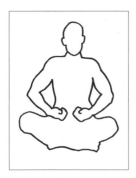

Ramona came for massages because they raised her mood so much. "And," she said, "there are no negative side effects!" I would massage down along her spine, and also along the inner edges of the bottoms of her feet. Then I taught her the cheerfulness mudra to use between appointments. It worked so well for her that she came for massages less often.

You can create your own cheerfulness. This mudra raises your mood, much like breathing in the scent of lavender does.

How to do it:
- Sit straight and tall.
- Put your hands on either side of your navel, palms up, fingers facing each other.
- With each hand, make a fist with your thumb inside.
- Relax your shoulders.
- Breathe deeply and slowly for 3 minutes.

Special note:
A couple of clients have said they get a build-up of too much energy in their thumbs when they do this mudra. Stick thumbs out between your index finger and middle finger to make it slightly less powerful.

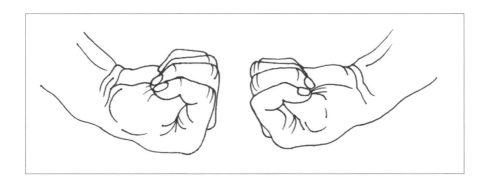

16 Self-confidence: Project positive energy

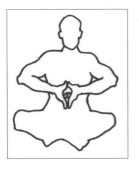

Julie had just started a new job. She said she knew she was good at what she did but she still felt very uneasy. I suggested she try the self-confidence mudra. We spent a couple of minutes doing it together, before her massage. I ran into her a couple of weeks later and she exclaimed that the mudra had really helped.

This mudra changes your perceptions, moving them in a more positive direction.

How to do it:
- Sit straight and tall.
- Press the pads of your index fingers together. Press the pads of your thumbs together. Curl your other fingers inward and let them touch, too. Place your hands on your belly, your thumbs just below your breast bone, your index fingers pointing out. You've now made an arrow pointing out.
- Breathe deeply and slowly for 3 minutes.

Special note:
This mudra can put you in touch with your own power.

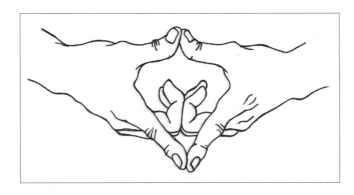

17 Prosperity: Live with abundance

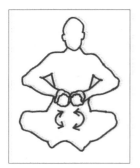

Norma had lost her job, so I taught her the prosperity mudra. She said, "I did the mudra everyday. Why not? I had nothing to lose. When I practiced the act of receiving, by making my hands into a bowl, I felt more like I deserved to receive. Practicing the mudra made me aware of opportunities I would have missed before. Now that I have a new job, I teach this to anyone willing to use it."

Prosperity is the ability to get what you need and want. With this mudra you take in what you need and you pour out your contribution. Doing this sets your intention.

How to do it:
- Sit straight and tall.
- Cup your hands, palms up with little fingers touching to form a bowl, symbolizing willingness to receive.
- Next turn palms over touching index fingers of your cupped hands together, emptying your bowl so you can recieve more.
- Breathe in when your bowl is right side up. Breathe out when your bowl is upside down.
- Repeat for 3 minutes.

Special note:
Imagine something pouring into and out of your bowl. Choose something that interests you – seeds, coins, candies, etc.

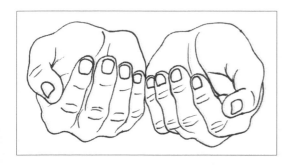

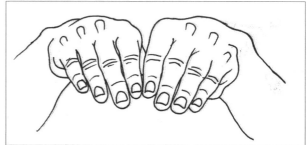

18 Courage: Release fear

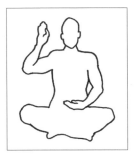

Natasha was afraid of her own shadow. She said this mudra helped her feel strong and more able to stand up for herself. She said, "I see my upraised hand as a stop sign. Don't come any closer! My bowl-shaped hand is asking for strength. I have the strength I need when I remember to ask for it. The deep breathing helps me feel strong, too."

Some say, with this mudra, you are asking for protection from whomever you put your faith in, which will vary according to your faith tradition. Sometimes when we're afraid we may attract what we fear. This mudra increases your courage.

How to do it:
- Sit straight and tall.
- Raise your right hand with your elbow bent, palm facing outward with fingers and thumbs straight up.
- Hold your left hand in front of your navel with the palm up.
  (Right hand asks for help. Left hand accepts the help.)
- Breathe deeply and slowly for 3 minutes. Inhale protection, exhale defeat.

Special note:
Affirm "I feel safe and protected."

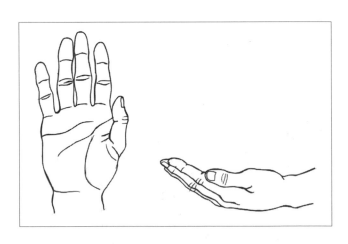

19 Vision: Clarify dreams and needs

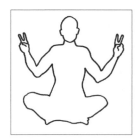

When I asked Kyra what she wanted from her massage, she said, "I've got this great plan for a new garden, and now I have to find the energy and motivation to actually do it!" After I gave her a massage, I taught her the vision mudra. She said, "Wow, I can hardly wait to get started on my garden. I know exactly what I will do." She left with a smile and fresh energy for her project.

Many people find this mudra energizing. Vision gives us the courage to get started and carry through.

How to do it:
- Sit straight and tall.
- Hold hands upright at ear level, palms facing forward.
- Place the tip of the thumb, ring finger, and little finger of each hand together to form a circle. Extend the other fingers.
- Breathe deeply and slowly for 3 minutes.

Special note:
This mudra helps to change your perception of what is possible. It helps you clarify your dreams, needs, and desires.

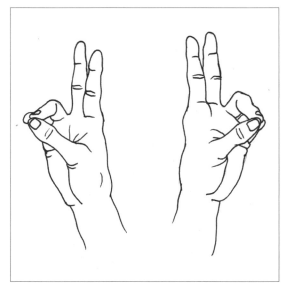

20 Overcome obstacles: Open the way for positive energy

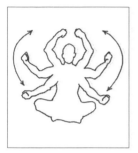

Amber was trying to make some major changes in her life. When she thought that she herself was getting in her own way, I taught her this mudra. After doing this mudra with me, she said, "This mudra makes me feel more effective. I'm clearing out my own mental obstacles, and now I have space where something new can grow."

This mudra helps you keep a positive outlook when facing difficulties.

How to do it:
• Sit straight and tall.
• Make fists with both hands, thumbs outside. Let your arms hang down and slightly behind you.
• Breathe in as you swing your arms up over your head, slightly forward. Breathe out as you swing your arms down.
• Proceed at your own pace for 3 minutes.

Special note:
This mudra should give you a feeling of power. If it doesn't, change how you are doing it a little. Try it standing up, with your feet a shoulder width apart, knees slightly bent.

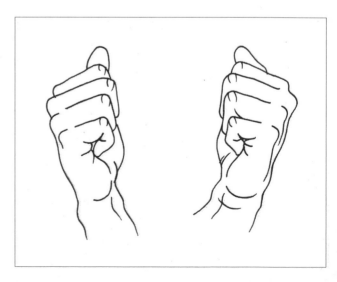

21 Balance: Reduce stress

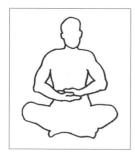

Barbara, a neighbor, complained about severe test anxiety. After giving her a calming massage, I offered to teach her a mudra for concentration. Just after placing her hands, one on top of the other, she smiled and said, "Oh! I get it!"

Later, she told me it really helped her study. And that by the end of the week, she only had to think about doing it, and she would be calm and focused. Every time anyone in my family runs into her, she says, "Tell Emily thank you so much for teaching me that mudra!"

When you are stressed, you are off center. You cannot hear your internal voice of wisdom. This mudra helps you slow down, concentrate, and center yourself.

How to do it:
- Sit straight and tall.
- Rest the back of the left hand in the palm of the right hand.
- Keep fingers together.
- Rest your hands on your belly, palms up, thumbs touching.
- Breathe deeply and slowly for 3 minutes.

Special note:
This mudra is the reverse of the forgiveness mudra. With balance the left hand is on top of the right. With forgiveness they are reversed. If you feel nothing, reverse hands to see if it helps. If you still feel nothing, try the focus mudra.

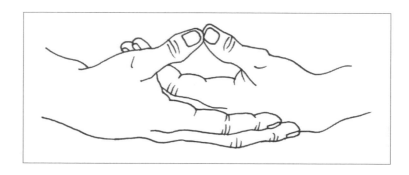

22 Memory: Increase mental power

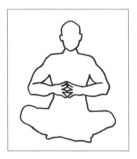

I met Chuck on an airplane and we started to talk about mudras. I was showing him the mudra for memory, and he said, "Wow! I do that all the time! My co-workers tease me about it, but I have a really good memory."

This mudra helps you concentrate, remember, and use both sides of your brain at once.

How to do it:
• Sit straight and tall.
• Press your fingertips together.
• Hold your thumbs just below your breastbone, but not touching your body. Other fingers are splayed outward.
• Breathe deeply and slowly for 3 minutes.

Special note:
Try putting your hands in front of your face with the points of your index fingers right between your eyebrows.

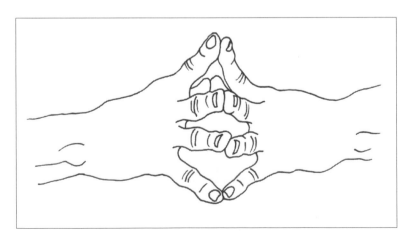

23 Clarity: Make clear decisions

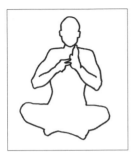

I showed this mudra to Glenda, a college student. She looked at me in astonishment and said, "I already do this mudra with the exact fingering you are using. I do it all the time when I'm studying, but I just thought I was fooling around!"

Clarity reduces mental fog and helps you make up your mind – especially when faced with important decisions.

How to do it:
- Sit straight and tall.
- Hold your left hand upright in a clapping position.
- Start at the base of your left palm. Slowly walk the index and middle fingers of your right hand up the palm of your left hand. Continue walking up the middle and ring fingers. When you get to the top of your left hand slowly walk the right hand back down.
- Repeat the walk up and down several times.
- Breathe deeply and slowly.

Special note:
If you are left handed, you might want to switch hands.

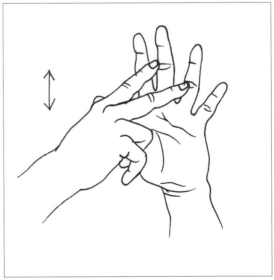

24 Focus: Increase calm and concentration

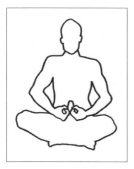

Kameka said, "When I do this mudra, everything extraneous falls away. I can think about one thing at a time. Usually my mind is all over the place, even when I take a test. It also really relaxes me, just like playing with sand does."

Focus reduces the distractions (clutter and chaos) of your mind and helps you concentrate on one issue.

How to do it:
- Sit straight and tall.
- Bring your hands together, palms up.
- Touch the backs of your fingers together.
- Make a circle with the thumbs and index fingers of each hand, with the index fingers resting lightly under the thumbs.
- Keep the other fingers straight up and touching.
- Rest hands on belly.
- Breathe deeply and slowly for 3 minutes.

Special note:
If this hand position is too difficult, try the balance mudra.

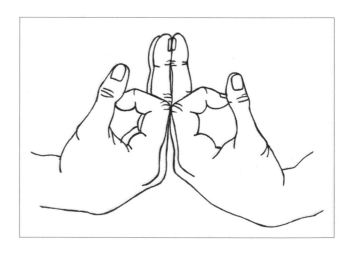

We have just looked at 24 mudras to release, relax, restore, recharge, reframe thinking, and refresh mind. In the next section we will look at ways these mudras can be combined to deal with several common situations.

Alphabetic Index of Mudras

Part Three:
Identifying What You Are Feeling

Types of feelings • How do I know what I am feeling?
Seven feeling poems • Tuning in to your feelings
How do I know if a feeling has a physical or emotional origin?

Identifying What You Are Feeling

When Cathy Lynn first came to me for massage, at the suggestion of her therapist, she had many stress symptoms. We talked briefly about what was going on in her life, and I could sense that she was unconnected to her feelings. She reported that people would say to her, "You must feel really angry about that," and she would assure them that no, she wasn't feeling any anger at all. Now she says, "But of course I was angry. I just didn't recognize my feelings." When Cathy learned to identify and release a number of her feelings, her stress-related symptoms disappeared.

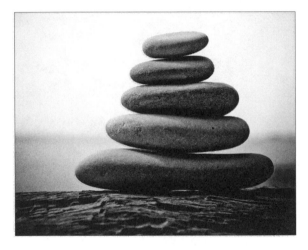

Just as Cathy had trouble dealing with her stress symptoms until she learned to recognize feelings, you may face the same problem. Once you have identified your feelings, you can choose strategies to help cope with them. Strategies could include mudras, massage, yoga, meditation, positive self-talk, journaling, writing poetry, playing or listening to music, dancing, other exercise, etc. Being able to identify feelings and then choose strategies to handle them should increase your sense of well-being.

In this chapter we will look at how people identify their feelings, and then present a procedure you can use to identify your feelings.

✋ Types of feelings: physical and emotional

Feelings – or sensations – can have physical origins or emotional origins. You can feel physical pain when you cut yourself, or emotional pain when someone is nasty toward you. Emotional distress can also cause physical pain in the body.

Stomach upset
Physical: Eating too much, or a food or drink that disagrees with you
Emotional: Anxiety or worries

My stomach feels upset if I'm about to speak before a large group of people I don't know. I therefore do not eat much before a presentation. Many people have this same experience.

Headache
Physical: Cheese, wine, chocolate – these and other foods can be triggers for a physical headache.
Emotional: Stress or anger can be a trigger for an emotional headache.

The worst headache I have ever had started at a wedding I attended a week before my own marriage. Watching all the attention focused on the bride intimidated me and stressed me out.

Fatigue or tiredness
Physical: Not enough sleep. Or, too much physical exertion: you have just helped move a friend from one apartment to another, or spent a whole day working in your yard, or all day on your feet with no breaks.

Emotional: You have spent several hours with a negative or critical person, or a child with a challenging temperament.

There are people in my life who have a lot of negative, critical energy. When I am around them much, I feel exhausted, regardless of my activities.

✋ How do I know what I'm feeling?

Begin with what you already know. In the exercise below are seven feelings to start with. Jot down any clues or things you discover about yourself.

Exercise: I know I'm Feeling *Something* When…

I know I'm feeling *happy* when:

I know I'm feeling *sad* when:

I know I'm feeling *angry* when:

I know I'm feeling *fear* when:

I know I'm feeling *anxiety* when:

I know I'm feeling *love* when:

I know I'm feeling *contentment* when:

Once you have jotted down your observations, look at the thoughts others had in the seven feeling poems below. Don't worry if your experiences are different from those expressed in the poems. Everyone experiences emotions in his or her own way.

✋ Seven feeling poems

I asked many people, "How do you know what you are feeling?" Here are some of the answers I received. I hope these poems help you become more aware of what you are feeling.

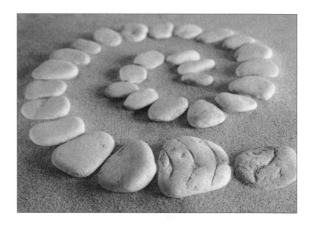

Happy
I feel light-hearted
And playful
There's a spring in my step
I breathe deeply
Wanting to hum or sing
Soft feelings fill my heart

Sad
I feel constricted in my chest
It's difficult to take deep breaths
Like I'm walking through molasses
My arms feel heavy
Tired and wilted
Tears come easily

Angry
I feel red hot or ice cold
My jaw starts to hurt
My heart beats faster
My feelings grow intense
I walk faster, talk faster, get louder
My body is rigid

Fear
My breathing gets shallow
There's a tightness in my belly
My voice gets squeaky
My motions get jerky
My muscles knot up
I feel cold, chilly

Love
I smile easily
Walk smoothly
My features soften
My heart feels open
I see the best in others
And feel connected

Contentment
I feel satisfied
My belly's relaxed
There is enough
For today and for tomorrow
My mood is pleasant
I enjoy just being

Anxiety/Worry
I can't eat or sleep
My muscles are tense
My movements are jerky
My mind dances around
Like a hummingbird
Thinking thoughts over and over

Some of these clues may resonate with you; perhaps you stop and think, "Yes! My heart does beat faster sometimes. I wonder if I might be angry when it does." If nothing resonates, that's fine. It means that you need to be your own detective and discover other clues to your feelings.

Tuning in to your feelings

Below is a process you can use to become aware of your feelings. When you begin to use this process it may feel awkward, but continue and it will get easier as you use it.

First, take three deep breaths. The deep breaths will help you tune in to yourself. You may be better able to recognize what you have been feeling when you are calmer. (see page 77 on "How to breathe with awareness.")

Second, ask, "What is going on inside my body right now?" Jot down a couple of words about what you notice as you tune in to each part.

• What does your head feel like?
• What does your neck feel like?
• What do your shoulders feel like?
• What does your heart feel like?
• What does your stomach feel like?
• What do your hands feel like?
• What do your feet feel like?

Third, what were you thinking about when you started to have this sensation? For some of us, certain thoughts habitually take us to a specific feeling state. For example, Christine's stomach hurts and her heart starts beating faster whenever she believes she is being ignored. Tom's jaw starts to hurt when he sees someone driving recklessly and endangering others.

Fourth, is there a physical reason for how you are feeling? When I start feeling grumpy, I need to ask myself:

- When did I last eat? Am I hungry?
- How much sleep have I been getting? Am I tired?
- When did I last go to the bathroom? Do I need to? (Some people get impatient without knowing why when they have to use the bathroom.)

Fifth, reflect on what you are feeling. When have you had similar thoughts and sensations, and what were you feeling then? Do any of your thoughts or sensations remind you of feelings in the poems? You may want to write some of your ideas down so you can come back later and compare how you feel at other times.

For example, when I jab at a computer key over and over, I know I am impatient and need to do the patience mudra so I can wait for the computer to respond.

What Am I Feeling: Step-by-Step	
Situation: Marie just left a meeting and is feeling awful.	
Steps	**Example**
1. **Take three deep breaths** in and out through your nose to center yourself, or in through nose and out through mouth.	*Why am I feeling so awful? What am I feeling? Breath. Breath. Breath.*
2. **What is going on inside your body now?** head? neck? shoulders? heart? stomach? hands? feet?	*My stomach feels tight and heavy. My shoulders are really stiff — almost like concrete.*
3. **What were you thinking about when the sensation started?** Sometimes thoughts habitually take us to a specific feeling state.	*I prepared an excellent presentation and they were not listening. They wanted me gone, one way or another. They were nasty.*
4. **Is there a reason for how you are feeling?** When did I last eat? How much sleep have I been getting? When did I last use the bathroom?	*I was fine before the meeting. I got enough sleep and I had a light lunch.*
5. **Reflect on what you are feeling.** When have you had similar thoughts and sensations, and what were you feeling? Do any of your thoughts or sensations remind you of feelings in the poems?	*The last time my stomach felt this bad, my new dog and I were being chased by a herd of angry cows and I was really scared. I guess I was feeling attacked by the committee and felt scared.*

✋ How do I know if a feeling has a physical or an emotional origin?

Physical and emotional sensations may be interlinked, so it can be hard to sort them out. You can feel tired because you are depressed. You can feel tired because you didn't get enough sleep. You might not be getting enough sleep because you are depressed. The reason you want to know whether a sensation is of physical or emotional origin is that the answer tells you where to start to make changes.

Sort out your sensations by starting with an emotional check-in and then go on to a physical check-in.

Emotional check-in
- What's going on inside of me? Has something been bothering me lately? Is there a recurring irritant or thought?
- What's going on around me? Angry people? People getting laid off at work? National politics depressing?
- What's going on in my circumstances or surroundings? Death/divorce/new job? Is my living space conducive to feeling good? Or is it cluttered and adding to my stress?

Physical check-in
- Am I getting enough sleep? Is lack of sleep causing me problems, or to respond emotionally in a way I wouldn't if my needs were met?
- Am I hungry? Am I eating regular meals each day?
- Is the food nutritious?
- Is my stress level way up?
- Am I getting enough exercise?

If you are not certain if your feeling is primarily physical or emotional, just start somewhere! Physically taking care of yourself by getting proper food, sleep, and exercise will help your emotional state. Working on your emotional state by deep breathing, medita-

tion, and mudras will also help your physical state. (I have meditated on the plane when I couldn't sleep, and actually felt like I *had* slept.)

Parents of small children often feel angry with their children not because of what their children have done but because the parents have not had their needs for proper food, sleep, or exercise met. When you fix one side of the equation, the physical or the emotional, it is likely to help the other, too.

We have looked at how physical and emotional sensations are linked and how they give us clues to what we are feeling. Once you know what you are feeling, it is easier to change unwanted feelings.

Once Cathy Lynn (story at the beginning of the chapter) could identify some of her feelings, she could work with me to release them. She had to be aware of them before she could release them. As she became aware of and able to express her feelings, most of her stress-related symptoms disappeared.

If you have trouble identifying your feelings, you can ask a trusted friend or professional what they think you might be feeling, or you can experiment with different mudras to see if there is an improvement.

When you have identified a feeling you want to release, you can either turn to chapter two and experiment with individual mudras, or go to chapter four and combine mudras to increase your sense of well-being.

Part Four:

Combining Mudras to Solve Issues

Common issues • How can I combine mudras myself?
Review • Step-by-step techniques • Sample worksheets

Combining Mudras to Solve Issues

Can mudras be combined and used to deal with common situations? Yes! Single mudras are useful. And, they can be combined to create even more powerful results. Below are several examples of how they have been combined. You may have to work with several mudras to get the changes you want. Let's see how this process works.

Common issues

Anger

Possible mudras: patience, cheerfulness, self-confidence
Imagine that you find it hard to manage your anger when dealing with your kids. (Many parents say, "I never lost my temper before I had kids!") You have a teenager who is very unhappy with you and knows how to push your buttons. He wants to use your car, but you have said no because he broke an agreement. You know that rather than raising your voice and getting ugly, you need to remain pleasant and remind him that he needs to find his own transportation.

Begin with a mudra to prevent anger. You might want to use the *patience* mudra or the *cheerfulness* mudra. Both of these help you stay calm. With the patience mudra, you can watch what's happening, but not get hooked. Doing the cheerfulness mudra, with your fingers wrapped around your thumbs, you feel surrounded by a protective cloak.

Before the actual confrontation, if you see it coming, do the *self-confidence* mudra. You will feel stronger and more energized. Afterward, do the *energy* mudra or, if your mind feels agitated, the *balance* mudra, to feel calm and centered.

After getting angry, when you are by yourself, try a release mudra, such as *release intense feelings,* where you pull feelings out of yourself and flick them away. If that offers you no relief, try the *calmness* mudra, where tensions are released through your arms.

Sometimes anger is legitimate — such as when your boundaries are being violated. When this is the case, you may want to explain your position and your expectation to resolve the situation.

Sometimes we take our frustrations out on other people. If you feel that you simply lost control, try the *self-forgiveness* mudra. Self-forgiveness isn't a thought, it's an action. It's something you do. If self-forgiveness is not your issue, try the *patience* mudra. This will help you get to a place where you can restore yourself.

Finally, do the *overcome obstacles* mudra. This mudra helps you change your perception. It helps you let go of obstacles that exist in your mind.

Money

Possible mudras: calming, tranquility, and prosperity
Suppose that you've been feeling some scarcity lately. There's been more going out of your bank account than has been coming in. There is just not enough money. You are feeling anxious. You start by releasing some of your anxiety so you won't feel so overwhelmed. You do the *calmness* mudra. It really does calm you. The knots that were in your stomach are gone. Do this mudra whenever you feel those knots in your stomach.

Now that you have released some of your anxious feelings, you want to concentrate on becoming really relaxed. Try the *tranquility* mudra, which will ground you and leave you with a quieter mind.

Next, you will do a reframe thinking mudra: the *prosperity* mudra, which will help you change your perceptions and be ready for new opportunities. Breathing in, from deep in your belly, you hold your hands like a bowl, so prosperity can flow in. Breathing out, you turn your hands over, emptying your bowl to share your energy, so you will have room to take more in.

Work-related

Possible mudras: release chaos, vision, clarity
Imagine that work is driving you crazy. You don't feel supported there currently, and you think about it all the time. It feels like your head is going to explode, and you don't know what to do.

First, pull gently on your ears to let out the tension in your head. This is the *release chaos* mudra. Next, do a reframe thinking mudra, called the *vision* mudra, to help you see things with new eyes and to give you a fresh start.

Last, do the *clarity* mudra to refresh your mind and make new learning easier. This mudra makes decisions clearer.

Loss of job

Possible mudras: self-confidence, prosperity, balance
Suppose that you have just lost your job. You've been laid off and you feel awful. You may be experiencing grief and anger, both of which you will need to deal with. But you also have to psych yourself up to go job hunting. Your self-esteem needs a boost. Start by doing the *self-confidence* mudra, to charge yourself up with positive energy and send it out into

the world. This can really give your morale a boost. Then use a reframe thinking mudra, the *prosperity* mudra. Some people say they feel more positive after doing this one and that they are more likely to see an event as an opportunity.

Your next mudra will be the *balance* mudra, which is in the refresh mind category. This will quiet the mind and help you stay centered and focused as you hunt for that new job.

Grief, sadness, and loss

Possible mudras: release intense feelings, tranquility, comfort
Suppose that you have just experienced the loss of someone close and you are feeling very sad. You want to combine mudras to change how you feel. It's not that you expect the grief to disappear (because it won't). But you want to lessen it enough that you don't feel overwhelmed or paralyzed.

Try the *releasing intense feelings* mudra first, where you pull some of that grief out of yourself and flick it away. If you are not aware of any relief from this mudra, try the *calming* mudra next. One of the places grief resides is in the forearms, so this mudra can help release it.

Next, do the *tranquility* mudra, which is a very relaxing mudra. Note that you are working with your forearms again. When you are feeling better, do a restoring mudra such as the *comfort* mudra, or the *cheerfulness* mudra to raise your mood. Remember to take deep, long breaths.

End of relationship

Possible mudras: comfort, contentment

Suppose that you have been in a relationship that has just ended, and you feel devastated. You just want to pull the blankets over your head and stay in bed. You feel like somehow you lost yourself in the relationship and you want your old self back – the one who liked being you and felt competent.

First, do the *comfort* mudra from the restore category. Your heart is aching, quite literally, and you need to treat it gently. Put your hands on your upper chest and send your heart soft, gentle, loving energy. Notice that you are soaking up the warmth from your own hands. Take long and deep breaths. You start to feel better.

Next, do another mudra from the restore category, the *contentment* mudra. Before you do it, release any hurtful thoughts of the past with the *release intense feelings* mudra. Contentment puts you in the present moment. You feel a friendship with yourself. Remember to take long, slow, deep breaths. You start to feel even better!

 ## How can I combine mudras myself?

The mudra wheel on page 67 can help you.

How can the mudra wheel help?

The mudra wheel makes it easier to use the mudras. It helps by organizing the mudras and offering a sequence which works for many people. The clockwise sequence is based on what I have found works well in massage. Release is a good place to start, but if you don't need to deal with feelings yet, you can skip it.

Some people might want to start around the wheel with refresh mind. If your mind is what you first engage in a crisis, refresh mind may be where you want to start. I usually need to deal with my feelings first. When I've dealt with my feelings, then I can think. Some people think first, and then they are ready to deal with their feelings.

If you choose a mudra, and get no results, you may need to do a mudra in the group before it (counterclockwise). For example, it's hard to receive feelings of comfort or contentment when you are not relaxed.

Combining mudras is like housekeeping, as you clear out the old stuff, you restore order, dust top to bottom, and open the windows.

 ## Review

Following is a review of the categories and questions that will help you choose between categories.

- *Release.* Mudras in the release group help you let go of strong feelings. They are active and intentional.

- *Relax.* Mudras in this group help you detach from concerns, and allow a sense of calm and peace to enter. They are passive and receptive.

- *Restore.* These mudras intentionally bring in new feelings. People often choose to invite feelings of love, comfort, and happiness.

- *Recharge.* Recharge mudras bring in energy. They banish discouragement and depression.

- *Reframe thinking.* Reframe mudras help people change their view of the world and how it operates.

- *Refresh mind.* The refresh mudras help the mind function. They either sharpen or quiet the mind.

Questions to guide you

Combining mudras is a process you can learn. It is not magic, and you can do it for yourself. Mudras are the tools. You can find out more about your feelings by asking the following questions:

- *"What do I need most?* Are my feelings over-whelming or too intense?"* If so, you'll do a *release* mudra.

- *"Am I feeling like fighting or running away?* Do I need to get out of the attack or being attacked mode?"* If so, you'll start with a *relax* mudra.

- *"Am I feeling disconnected and lonely?* Do I need nurturing? Do I feel in need of comfort, contentment, happiness, or love?"* If so, you'll do a *restore* mudra.

- *"Do I feel underfunded with either energy or enthusiasm?* Do I need to energize myself, perhaps with cheerfulness or self-confidence?"* If so, you'll do a *recharge* mudra.

- *"Am I a victim of my own negative thoughts, especially of the 'I can't do that' variety? As in, 'I can't write a book, release my fears, finish my schooling,' etc.?"* If so, you'll do a *reframe thinking* mudra.

- *"Do I have trouble studying or learning because I can't think of just one thing at a time? Is my mind all over the place? Do I need more clarity or focus?"* If so, you'll do a *refresh mind* mudra.

To combine mudras, you need to decide what is most important. What functions of the mudra wheel do you need most? Are there some that you don't need at all right now? When you first start combining mudras, limit yourself to three or four.

In this section we looked at several examples of how mudras can be combined, and then we looked at how you can combine them yourself using the mudra wheel on page 67. The next section shows a process you can use to make them a part of your life. Without a plan, good intentions tend to fizzle. Now that you know what you want to do, this section shows you *how* to do it.

Mudra Wheel

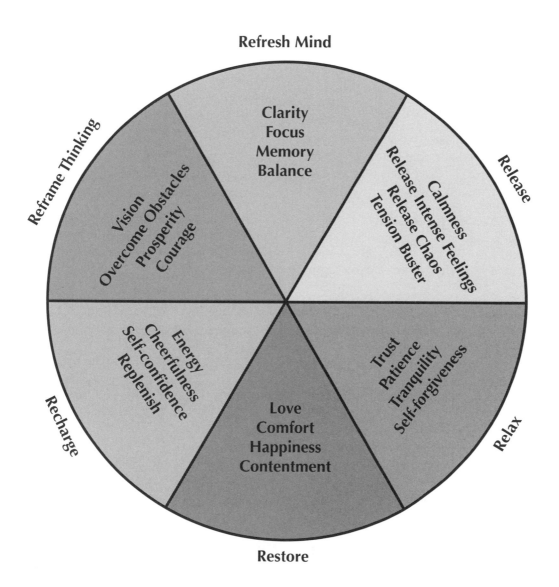

Refresh Mind

Clarity
Focus
Memory
Balance

Release

Calmness
Release Intense Feelings
Release Chaos
Tension Buster

Reframe Thinking

Vision
Overcome Obstacles
Prosperity
Courage

Relax

Trust
Patience
Tranquility
Self-forgiveness

Recharge

Energy
Cheerfulness
Self-confidence
Replenish

Restore

Love
Comfort
Happiness
Contentment

Step-by-step techniques

Are you ready to work with mudras to create changes in your life? If you are, but need structure, here is a process to help you get started. On the following pages there are four sample work sheets, and a fifth, which is blank, for you to use.

1 Stop and focus

Before you change something, you have to know what you want to change. It could be issues with money, memory, clutter, or relationships. Think of one thing you complained about last week. Write a sentence about how your life would be different if this issue were solved.

2 Think of mudra-related ideas

What mudras do you think might help you with your issue? Is there a category of mudras you want to look at, for example, recharge mudras if you have a lack of energy?

3 Think of other ideas that might help you

If you are having trouble sleeping, generate ideas you might want to try, such as drinking chamomile tea in the evenings, avoiding exercise or bright lights close to bedtime, and so on.

4 Choose an action

What mudras are you actually going to do? What supporting actions are you going to do? Write down what you are going to do and when you are going to do it. Will you do it in the morning when you first wake up? Right before you go to bed? Write down how you are going to remember to do it. You can post reminders on your bathroom mirror, or leave mudra reminders on the answering machine. How long are you going to do it? Two weeks?

One month? Now that you have decided what you will do, take control and do it.

5 Review, revise, and reward

When reviewing, you need to stop and focus. Has anything changed? If not, you need to think of some mudra-related ideas. Do you need to do your mudras more frequently? Do you need to switch to different mudras? Now think of some other ideas, *not* mudra related. For example, you could get window shades that block sunlight if you are trying to improve your sleep. Whatever you decide to do, it is important to think about when to do it, how you will remember to do it, and how long to do it.

If your plan is working well and you have achieved your goal, celebrate! You deserve it! What I would do, of course, is go out and have tea with a friend. How would you celebrate? When we honor our successes by acknowledging them, we are setting ourselves up for more success.

 Sample worksheets

The following is a worksheet of the step-by-step process above. To make it even easier to follow, four samples of how to use it with different issues are provided.

Sample 1: Relationship Anxiety	
Situation: Lydia's complaint was not having a relationship.	
Steps	**Examples**
Stop and focus: What do I want? What is my vision?	I want a relationship – • which feels right. • in which I feel respected. • where I don't feel like I have to give up myself to make it work. • where there's room for us each to have separate activities.
How would my life be different without this issue?	• I would have a relationship based on trust and respect.
Think of ideas: What mudras could help me?	I could – • do the *overcoming obstacles* mudra, to help me change my belief that there's no one out there right for me. • do the *clarity* mudra, to help me with discernment.
Generate other ideas	I could – • join groups that do things I love to do as a way of meeting new people. • ask friends to introduce me to their friends.
Act effectively: Make a plan	I will – • do the *overcoming obstacles* mudra first thing in the morning. • tape a reminder to do it on the refrigerator. • keep the *clarity* mudra card on my night stand. • When I do the *clarity* mudra, I will say to myself, "My discernment improves every day."
Remove roadblocks	The *overcoming obstacles* mudra is for releasing the obstacle of my negative thinking.
Review, revise and celebrate	In four weeks time I will reflect on whether I see any changes in my attitudes or in my discernment. • If I see no changes, I may want to do the mudras for a longer period of time, or more frequently. • I could also try different mudras. If I do see changes in my thinking, I will celebrate by taking a long walk with a friend!

Sample 2: Too Much Clutter	

Situation: Kathy didn't like having people over because of her clutter, especially in the living room. She had plastic bags and boxes with stuff in them that she never got around to sorting.

Steps	Examples
Stop and focus: What do I want? What is my vision?	• I want control of my clutter. • I want balance: if I want new stuff, I have to get rid of old stuff. No input without output.
How would my life be different without this issue?	• My living room would be neat. • It would convey a feeling of welcome and comfort to family and friends.
Think of ideas: What mudras could help me?	I could do the – • *prosperity* mudra because it models letting go before taking in. • *balance* mudra to help me when sorting.
Generate other ideas	I could – • read a book on decluttering. • find myself a clutter buddy for mutual support • do a three-pile sort: keep, give away, and throw out. • set a time for getting rid of stuff that I truly dislike.
Act effectively: Make a plan	I will – • practice the *prosperity* mudra in the morning and before bed. • do the *balance* mudra for focus right before I start to sort and say, "I easily stay on task." • spend 20 minutes a day before noon sorting out my living room boxes. • set a timer when I start working on a clutter box, so I don't procrastinate because the task seems too large. • say "I easily release things I no longer need" often.
Remove roadblocks	I will collect the things I need, such as baskets, folders, magic markers, ahead of time.
Review, revise and celebrate	In one month, I will see if I think the mudras have helped: "Have I been able to focus and let go of significant clutter?" "Have I taken many bags to Goodwill?" • If so, this is success. I will celebrate by having friends over for tea to sit in front of the fireplace in my newly decluttered living room. • If not, I'll do the mudra longer, more often, or I can switch.

Sample 3: Fear of Aging

Situation: Ernesto caught himself saying over and over again: "I can't remember anything anymore." "I'm too young to be having 'senior moments'," or, "I'm afraid I'm getting old before my time."

Steps	Examples
Stop and focus: What do I want? What is my vision?	• I want to look at aging as a positive experience. • I need to find things to do that will help me feel confident. • I want to live without worrying about what I am forgetting.
How would my life be different without this issue?	• I would remember what I wanted, when I wanted it. • I would feel confident rather than apologetic. • If my memory improved, I would feel less stress.
Think of ideas: What mudras could help me?	• I could do the *memory* mudra to help me remember. • I could do the *self-confidence* mudra to increase my confidence in my memory.
Generate other ideas	I could: • read a book on positive aging or the aging brain. • do crossword puzzles to stimulate my brain. • ask my physician how to improve my memory. • take a supplement to improve circulation in the brain. • get more exercise to clear out my brain. • play computer games designed to increase mental strength (such as those on www.Luminosity.com).
Act effectively: Make a plan What will you do? When will you do it? How will you remember it?	• I will do the *self-confidence* mudra and the *memory* mudra every morning. • I'll start on Monday. • I will keep both mudra cards on my night stand to remind me to do them. • I will call Tuesday morning to schedule a physical and ask for suggestions to exercise my brain.
Remove roadblocks	Because I still might forget to do the mudras, I will put a sticky note on the bathroom mirror and one on my coffee machine.
Review, revise and celebrate	In one month — • I will see if I think the mudras have made any difference. • If I find, for example, that I don't have to walk downstairs to remember why I went upstairs, that's success!

Sample 4: Unemployment Anxiety

Situation: Nancy had been out of work for _____. She would apply for jobs but not get them. This resulted in a lack of self-confidence, which made her situation worse.

Steps	Examples
Stop and focus: What do I want? What is my vision?	• I want the confidence to believe that somebody out there will hire me. • I want a job that would use my skills and pay my bills with enough left over for savings and small luxuries.
How would my life be different without this issue?	• I would have an expectation that people would hire me. I'm a competent person and I have employable skills.
Think of ideas: What mudras could help me?	• The *self-confidence* mudra seems like a natural. Self-confidence is what's missing in my current job search. • The *prosperity* mudra might help me recognize opportunity where I have not seen it before.
Generate other ideas	• I have already gotten professional help from an employment counselor. • I have updated my resume and my appearance. • I believe I would benefit from some role-playing of an interviewing situation to get feedback on how I am presenting myself.
Act effectively: Make a plan	Starting Monday — • I will do both the *self-confidence* mudra and the *prosperity* mudra every day, morning and evening. • I will tape a note on my bathroom mirror to remind me to do them both in the morning before I start my day. • I will leave both mudra cards on the night stand next to my bed to remind me to do them in the evening. • When I do the *self-confidence* mudra, I will visualize a self-confident me, and I will say, "I gain confidence each day." • Each time I do the *prosperity* mudra I will visualize myself receiving something of value. • I will say to myself, "I have more than enough."
Remove roadblocks	I've chosen mudras to increase my energy and improve my attitude, which should in turn remove roadblocks.
Review, revise and celebrate	In two weeks time — • I will reflect on my mudra practice and whether I see any changes in my self-confidence and employment opportunities. • If I have found employment I need to celebrate. I will celebrate by inviting someone over for tea and scones.

We have just seen how the worksheet can be used to incorporate mudras into your daily life. Now I'm offering you a worksheet so you can work on your own concerns. There is a saying, "If you want to learn to cook, you must spend some time in the kitchen." This is your opportunity to head to the kitchen.

Worksheet for Your Issue	
Situation:	
Steps	**Examples**
Stop and focus: What do I want? What is my vision?	
How would my life be different without this issue?	
Think of ideas: What mudras could help?	
Generate other ideas	
Act effectively: Make a plan. What will you do? When will you do it? How will you remember it?	
Remove roadblocks	
Review, revise and celebrate	

In this chapter we have looked at how you can combine mudras and make a plan to meet your individual needs. In the next chapter we will look at ways you can enhance the power of the mudras.

Part Five:
Enhancing the Power of Mudras

Ways to strengthen mudras • Closing

Enhancing the Power of Mudras

There are several things you can do to enhance the effectiveness of mudras. First and foremost is breathing with awareness. Second, practice mudras consistently, for short periods of time. Third, create a friendly environment where you control the temperature, and remove clutter and other distractions. And fourth, you can engage all your senses (sight, sound, smell, taste, and touch) for a wonderful synergistic effect.

✋ Ways to strengthen mudras

Breathing
Why is breathing so important? It's how the body dispels tension. When you're stressed, the sympathetic nervous system is in charge of your body and your muscles are tense. You are "on alert," in a "fight or flight" pattern. When the parasympathetic nervous system is in charge of the body, it is no longer on alert. The body can relax.

Breathing is the key element that changes your physical and emotional state. When you breathe slowly and deeply the parasympathetic nervous system takes over. Just taking four deep, long, slow breaths starts the relaxation process.

During massage when I work on clients' shoulders, I ask them to take four deep, slow, long breaths. By the time they finish the four breaths, the muscles I'm working on have started to loosen up.

How to breathe with awareness
- *Get in a comfortable position* — Back straight; feet and arms uncrossed.
- *Begin breathing.* Start with your belly. To help, place a hand on your belly to fill it filling up. As you start to breathe, remember you are breathing in fresh air. (In with the *new*.) Keep breathing as your belly fills up, your chest expands, and your lungs fill up.
- *Pause.* When you can't breathe in any more air, be aware of your breath for just a moment.
- *Release breath.* When you let out the breath, you are releasing stale air. (Out with the *old*.) Your lungs start emptying out, your chest contracts, and then your belly feels empty.
- *Pause again.* Be aware of your empty belly for just a moment.
- *Start the cycle over* by breathing in fresh air. With a hand on your belly, feel it filling up.

Consistent practice
Why is consistent practice important? Because later when you need a mudra you can call on it. Mudras are a prompt for your body to respond in a certain way. The more you practice calming yourself, for example, the easier it will become. Like any new skill, it takes practice. You also need to be intentional and focused while you do mudras. You don't, for example, watch television or work on your to-do list at the same time. You need to be present and committed.

Create a friendly environment
Why is setting up the environment important? When we are surrounded by clutter, many of us can't breathe or concentrate. Clutter drains us and drags us down. We feel blah. I personally do best when my space is set up to help me do whatever I'm there to do. That's what I'm asking you to do. Have a mudra support corner in your house. It can be very small, just a shelf will do. It can be simple, a few objects that you like, placed there to help you focus.

Engage your senses
Why is engaging the senses important? Because, when you add another appropriate sensory element, you benefit from the synergy. What is synergy? It occurs when several things work together to create greater benefit than anything alone can.

Esther, who said she didn't know how to relax, ex-claimed, after a massage, "It's not the candle, the music, or the tea. It's not the lotion, the textures, or the touch. It's everything!" Every added sense increases the impact of the whole experience.

This enhancement is true for both massage and mudras. The key here is use of appropriate sensory elements. If you want to relax, you don't put on a rousing march and drink highly caffeinated beverages.

Let's take a relaxing journey through the senses. These are examples of what you can use to help yourself relax. You would make different choices to energize yourself.

Touch: Practice a relaxing mudra (*tranquility*) or play with sand.
Sound: Listen to the sound of ocean waves, or affirm out loud, "I am relaxed," or "Ocean waves relax me."
Sight: Gaze at a picture of waves or a goldfish bowl. Or, visualize yourself relaxed, floating on the water.
Taste: Drink chamomile tea, or eat toasted seaweed or dried apples.
Smell: Light a lavender or ocean-scented candle.

When you take care with your breathing and your environment, involve all your senses, and practice consistently, you are setting yourself up for success.

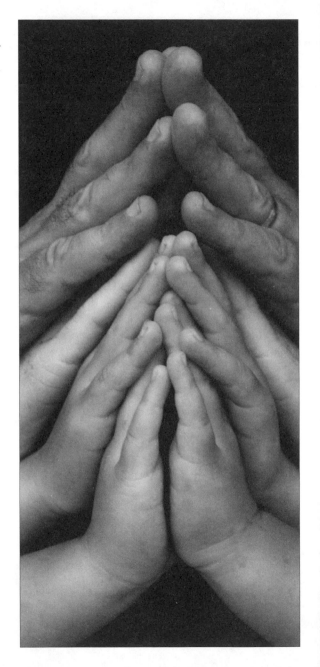

Closing

As you work with these mudras, they will become your friends. They will help you through whatever changes you decide to make. The mudra wheel shows six different ways to use them. You may combine mudras when you have more than one reason to use them.

You may enhance your mudras by consistent practice, breath awareness, setting the stage, and engaging your senses.

Remember, you can use mudras to great effect in the middle of your busy life. When conditions aren't perfect, adapt your mudra practice to them. For example, you can do many mudras quietly in your lap, while other people are present. Any place, any time, you can use a mudra like *balance* to quiet your mind. Breath awareness and the mudra are all you need. Once your mind is quiet, you are better able to deal with anything!

When life is challenging, be gentle with yourself by using mudras. As you experiment with what works, remember it takes practice to do mudras skillfully. As you do them more, they get easier. If practicing with others motivates you, find a mudra buddy. If you are having trouble getting started, make a plan.

When I first encountered mudras, I didn't know how to get started. I was motivated, but without any structure. I wrote this book to help you get started. I'm leaving you in good hands: your own.

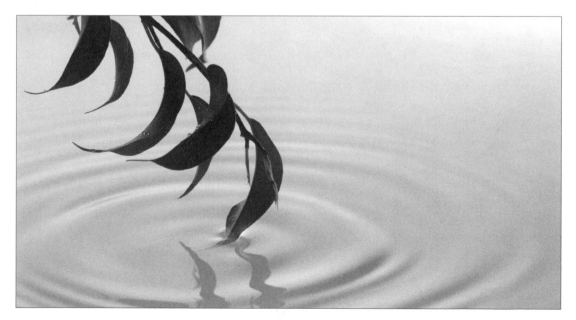

Resources

These items that may help you get into the right mind-set to practice mudras more easily.

Scents

Release
White sage and cedarwood cleanse and purify.
Relax
Lavender and chamomile are well known for their calming properties.
Restore
Green tea comforts, Rose heals grieving hearts.
Recharge
Ginger and cinnamon warm and energize.
Reframe thinking
Bergamot has been used to change mood or attitude.
Refresh mind
Rosemary and peppermint clarify thinking.

Many of these scents are available as a lotion, candle, or tea. They can be found at local grocery, drug and health food stores, and co-ops, and online. Check the ingredients list to be sure the product is up to your standard. My favorite places are:
www.AlohaBay.com
www.BathandBodynet.com
www.BathandBodyworks.com
www.CelestialSeasonings.com
www.harney.com
www.healinggarden.com
www.juniperridge.com
www.medicineflower.com
www.REPUBLICofTEA.com
www.revolutiontea.com.
www.trumelange.com

Music

Release
Migration by Carlos Nakai and Peter Kater, Native American Flute, 1992
Relax
Relaxation and Meditation with Music and Nature: Ocean Voyage by David Miles Huber, Laser Light Digital
Restore
The Mystic Harp by Derek Bell, Clarity Sound & Light
Recharge
The Memory of Trees by Enya
Reframe thinking
Relaxation and Meditation with Music and Nature: Distant Thunder by David Miles Huber
Refresh mind
Pachelbel: In the Garden by David Gibson's *Solitudes:* Exploring Nature with Music

Potpouri

Release
Burn White Sage Wild Incense, available at www.juniperridge.com.
Relax
Play with fine-grain sand.
Restore
Hold rose quartz.
Recharge
Play chimes or a singing bowl, available at www.tenthousandvillages.com.
Reframe thinking
Eat dark chocolate, stroke silk charmause fabric, or let flax seed drift between your fingers.
Refresh mind
Suck on peppermint candy, chew spearmint gum. Brush hair or pinch toes.

Books

Aromatherapy: A Complete Guide to the Healing Art,
2nd ed., by Kathi Keville. Berkeley, Calif.: Crossing Press,
2008.

The Deeper Dimensions of Yoga: Theory and Practice
by George Feuerstein. Boston: Shambhala, 2003.

*The Fine Arts of Relaxation, Concentration, and
Meditation: Ancient Skills for Modern Minds*, rev. ed.,
by Joel and Michelle Levey. Somerville, Mass.: Wisdom
Publications, 2003.

Healing Mudras: Yoga for Your Hands by Sabrina
Mesko. New York: Wellspring/Ballantine, 2000.

*Mudra: A Study of Symbolic Gestures in Japanese
Buddhist Sculpture* by E. Dale Saunders. Princeton, NJ:
Princeton University Press, 1960.

Mudras: Yoga in Your Hands by Gertrud Hirschi. San
Francisco: Red Wheel/Weiser, 2000.

Web Sites

Emily Fuller Williams, www.innerpeacemudras.com
Mudra card deck, www.ParentingPress.com, forthcoming

Index

Mudra Diary

About the Author

Emily Fuller Williams began her career in medical research and has been practicing massage therapy since the 1980s. Her training included the concepts of traditional Chinese medicine, with an emphasis on the emotional benefits of massage. Today she practices with a group of psychologists.

For the past several years, Williams has incorporated mudras into her practice. These ancient gestures, based on several Eastern traditions, can be done anywhere, any time. Within minutes they allow a person to release tension, relax muscles, and restore mental focus. Williams has taught the mudras in this book to people of all ages, including those who work in such physically and emotionally demanding professions as hospice, mental health, and teaching.

"People who listen, really listen to their bodies and then both reflect and respond to what their bodies are telling them have an exceptional opportunity to ease stress and improve well-being," Williams tells her clients and workshop participants.

A graduate of the University of Wisconsin at Madison, Williams lives in Cleveland, Ohio, with her husband and two sons.

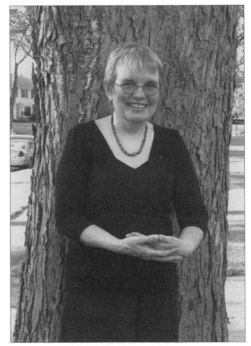